Prenatal Care

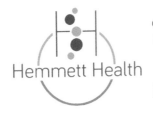

Find us on LinkedIn, Google+, Facebook and Instagram to learn more great health tips, get to know our providers and join the Hemmett Health family!

HemmettHealth.com
802-879-1703

Prenatal Care

EMPOWERMENT STRATEGIES FOR A VIBRANT PREGNANCY

Jeffrey —
To changing the
world!

It's just An
issue

Dr. Vicki Hemmett & Dr. Erik Hemmett
Chiropractic Physicians

With a Foreword by
Dr. Jane "Jennie" Lowell, OB-GYN
HemmettHealth.com

Empowering People to Live Happy, Healthy, and Vibrant Lives

ISBN: 0692749365
ISBN 13: 9780692749364
Library of Congress Control Number: 2016910613
Hemmett Health, South Burlington, VT

Contents

Illustrations

Foreword

I am a practicing ob-gyn physician at Maitri Health Care for Women in South Burlington, Vermont. I have been lucky enough to work with the exceptional team at Hemmett Health since 2008, when both of our practices moved to the Eastern View Integrated Medicine Center. Eastern View opened with the goal of establishing collaborative relationships between varying health care disciplines, in the hope of providing comprehensive and superior health care services to our clients. Hemmett Health's office is right across the hall from mine, and the proximity of our offices has promoted fantastic dialogue and communication, which has only enhanced our relationship and expanded the diversity of quality patient-care services offered. Since 2008, they have taught me quite a lot in terms of palpating and evaluating for musculoskeletal causes of pain—such as the psoas involvement in lower-quadrant pain and the pelvic floor muscles in a diversity of pelvic floor conditions and pain syndromes.

Over the years, I have come to have more experience with Hemmett Health's care. I have gained increased trust of and knowledge in their diverse services, and I now refer patients to them even more than I did when we first started our relationship. This is entirely because I see the results and improvements my patients have achieved after being seen at their practice. It is a joy to have the services of Hemmett Health to offer to my patients because I know they will see positive results.

As an ob-gyn, I refer my pregnant patients to Hemmett Health frequently for sacroiliac joint, lower-back, and hip pain and pubic symphysis. The patients are so happy to feel relief from their pain and to maintain their mobility without requiring prescription drugs. For patients with breech presentations, I refer them to Hemmett Health for a technique that Dr. Vicki has developed, which sometimes alone can vert a breech fetus or at least make the maternal abdomen more relaxed and my attempts at an external cephalic version more successful. I appreciate their comprehensive look at what is causing the pain and their focus on educating women about how to stretch and strengthen to proactively prevent problems from worsening or creeping up as their bodies change in pregnancy.

Postpartum, I now routinely assess my patients at six weeks for pelvic floor muscle dysfunction, whether it be hypotonia or hypertonia, and I send these women to Hemmett Health for the Hemmett pelvic floor release technique (HPFRT), which is a manual pelvic floor myofascial release technique that Dr. Vicki developed. Women suffering from dyspareunia, tailbone pain, and incontinence issues typically markedly improve or are normal after a limited numbers of treatment sessions. Most women feel much better within two visits, some of whom had been unsuccessfully treated for much longer periods of time elsewhere. The Hemmett office is also great about helping women rehabilitate their core muscles, which get so stretched out during pregnancy and childbirth. They have a great comprehensive postnatal program focused on strengthening and returning women's normal muscle function and tone (both abdominal and pelvic floor). This helps prevent future problems for these women, such as back pain and pelvic floor dysfunction.

I have had women present to me with complaints of years of pelvic pain and dyspareunia, and thanks to my work with Hemmett Health, I now know how to assess them for pelvic-floor-muscle sources of pain, in addition to my typical gynecologic work up. If I find a pelvic-floor-muscle component to patients' pain, I refer them to Hemmett Health, and I have seen people cured of their pain after years of suffering. I have had annual patients tell me they can't exercise because of their back, hip, or iliotibial band pain, and I have referred them to Hemmett Health for treatment, including active release techniques (ART). These patients return thanking me for the referral because they can now exercise again. My own father, a retired MD, called me in a panic with hip pain, thinking he should go to the ER because he hurt so much. I encouraged him to go to Hemmett Health, and they diagnosed and treated him for bursitis. I had a patient who showed up at my office in tears because she was in so much pain she thought she had a ruptured ovarian cyst. I quickly confirmed with ultrasound that she had normal gynecologic anatomy and palpated her psoas muscle (as Dr. Vicki had taught me to do) and realized that this muscle was in spasm and likely causing her pain. I walked her directly to the Hemmett Health office, where they evaluated and treated her. She left the building pain free one hour later.

I feel quite lucky professionally to have such skilled and gifted clinicians across the hall from me. My patients have benefited so much from their skills. I appreciate the quick and amazing results they get. I also appreciate that I can offer my patients treatment that is risk free, avoids narcotic prescriptions, is very cost effective, and is so comprehensive. The joy in

my job comes from being able to help people feel better, and since working with the Hemmetts, I have so much more that I can offer people to achieve this goal. That is a gift to me and to my patients.

Sincerely,
Jennie Lowell, MD
Maitri Health Care for Women
Eastern View Integrative Medicine
185 Tilley Drive
South Burlington, VT 05403

Introduction

Parenthood is one of the most wonderfully rewarding and challenging experiences in life, and with it come many changes, beginning during pregnancy. Pregnancy changes a woman's body in many different ways. Hormonal changes loosen all the body's ligaments, requiring muscles to work harder to stabilize joints, which can easily lead to overuse problems and pain. The laxity, coupled with healthy weight gain and changes in the center of gravity, contributes to common overuse pain syndromes. Foot, knee, pelvis, lower back, shoulder, head, and neck pain, as well as sciatica and tingling in the hands, can all be related to the changes in your growing body.

There are many safe, effective, and gentle home-based and conservative office techniques to relieve these pain syndromes. Soft-tissue techniques, including self-stretching, partner massage, and core-stabilization strengthening, in combination with a focus on ergonomics and modification of daily life activities, can make a huge difference in how you feel during your pregnancy and how well you recover after the birth. The key to preventing and alleviating common overuse syndromes associated with pregnancy is being strong, stable and flexible, while maintaining a neutral posture as much as possible.

Let us help you fully embrace your pregnancy by taking care of your changing body!

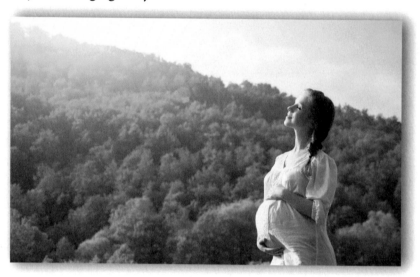

CHAPTER 1

Goal of This Book

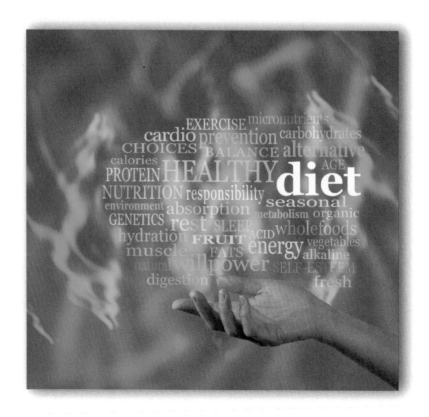

emmett Health published this book to be a valuable resource to empower every woman who is pregnant or planning to become pregnant. As well, we wrote this book to be used as a tool for anyone who cares about or loves a woman who is planning to get pregnant or is pregnant, to help her along her wonderful pregnancy journey.

We hope to help you learn how to properly prepare for pregnancy, manage your body throughout the journey, and give yourself the best chance of a successful recovery afterward. This book is intended to educate you about the most common conditions that arise and empower you with self-care techniques and an awareness of office-based therapies that are available to help you. In most cases, you do not need to live with pain throughout your pregnancy.

We will have three sequels to this book, covering postnatal care, pelvic floor care, and pediatric care (highlighting the most common repetitive strain injuries in kids). *Prenatal Care* will cover the planning phase of pregnancy through to the birth.

What Our Goal Is Not and Legal Disclaimer

This book is intended for educational purposes only. This book is not intended to diagnose or treat any illness. Diagnosis and treatment should be performed by a qualified member of your pregnancy health care team. You should not attempt these self-care protocols without the consent of one of your qualified health care team members. There are some very serious conditions that can mimic the conditions described in this book, and only a properly qualified health care professional can make that determination. Seek help immediately if you experience a severe onset of pain that is not relieved by anything or that lasts longer than twenty-four hours, as this may be a sign of a serious medical condition such as a blood clot.

CHAPTER 2

Team Health Care and Collaborative Medicine

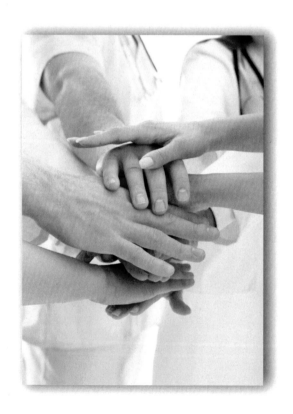

Who to Have on Your Prenatal Health Care Team

Health care is a team effort. Each health care provider is a team member with a special role. Some team members are doctors who help diagnose disease. Others are experts who treat disease or care for patients' physical and emotional needs. No one provider will have the solutions to all of your pregnancy health care needs.

Obstetrician, Primary Care Physician (PCP), Midwife, or Other Home-Birthing Provider

Your obstetrician, PCP, midwife, or other home-birthing provider is the center of the team. He or she should be aware of all the other providers you are seeing and should support your health care values. We encourage you to interview a couple of different providers and find the right person for you. Ask those you interview for their C-section rates, the number of deliveries they manage per year, and whether they have any concerns about the other team members you have or would like to assemble. This person will be with you throughout your pregnancy and will play an essential role during the birth.

Chiropractor

Chiropractors practice in many different ways. We encourage you to find one who has training in a soft-tissue therapy like the ones we recommend in chapter 9 ("Office-Based Care") as well as chiropractic joint manipulation and basic low-tech rehab exercises. The chiropractor should also encourage active patient participation with home exercises like stretching and mild functional-strengthening exercises. It is of additional benefit if your chiropractor is able to fit you for the type of custom orthotics that we recommend on the "Endorsed Products" page of HemmettHealth.com.

Rehabilitation Therapist: Physical Therapist, Licensed Athletic Trainer, or other

A rehabilitation therapist will work with your chiropractor and address muscular weakness or tightness as needed. He or she can provide training in posture, ergonomics, and biomechanics. A rehabilitation therapist may also practice soft-tissue techniques like the ones we recommend in chapter 9. Similar to your chiropractor, your therapist should offer a healthy balance of passive and active in-office care and active home-based care.

Nutritionist or Dietician

Nutrition is very important during pregnancy. This provider will advise you on the nutritional requirements for pregnancy and identify potential deficiencies you may have. Your nutritionist or dietician can also help you with meal preparation and planning.

Doula

A doula provides emotional, physical, and informational support during the time leading up to labor, during the birth itself, and immediately afterward. A doula has extensive knowledge of pregnancy and birth and provides a quiet, confident presence in the last weeks of your pregnancy, during the labor, and in the immediate weeks postpartum. A doula offers continuous support, staying beside you and your partner throughout the entire labor.

Massage Therapist

Massage therapy during pregnancy is a wonderful complementary therapy to prenatal care. It is a healthy way to reduce stress and promote overall wellness. Massage can help relieve many of the common discomforts experienced during pregnancy, such as low-back pain, neck and shoulder stiffness, hip pain, and edema (swelling). In addition, prenatal massage can reduce stress on weight-bearing joints, encourage blood and lymph circulation, help relax nervous tension (which may improve sleep), and help relieve depression or anxiety caused by hormonal changes.

It is best to seek out a therapist who is certified in or has experience with pregnancy massage. The therapist should know what is and is not safe for the mother and her baby, and he or she should have knowledge of pregnancy and the anatomy of a pregnant woman.

Your team needs to work together to safely protect, support, and guide you in achieving your prenatal goals. If you find that one of your team members refuses to participate with you or other providers on your health care team, then find a replacement. No one provider has the answer to all of your questions, concerns, and challenges. Make sure you are comfortable being honest and up front with all of your team members and that they provide excellent information about the options that are best supported by evidence or their clinical experiences while also taking your individual values into consideration. Not all therapy options in medicine align with all the values of the patient. Protect your right to choose which options are and are not appropriate for you.

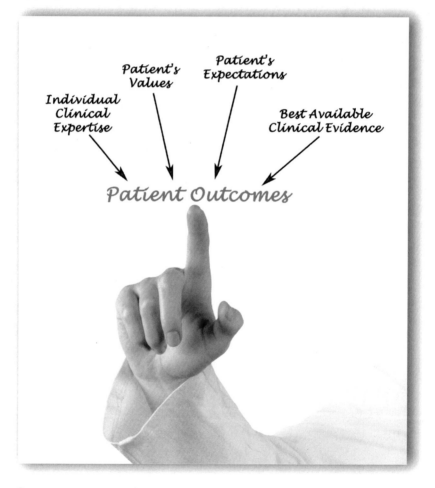

Evidence-Based Medicine

Evidence-based medicine gives equal weight to the best available research, the clinical experience of the provider, and the values of the patient. Increasingly, high-quality research evidence is the cornerstone of evidence-based health care decisions and is critically important to physicians, patients, policy makers, and payers. This data-driven evolution in decision making will impact health care in many ways. It should serve to level the playing field to allow all parties to be treated fairly and transparently and should ensure that patients can choose their providers for high-quality, cost-effective health care services.

On a larger scale, support those local, state, and federal legislators and policy makers who protect your right to choose which medical providers and treatments are or are not appropriate for your own values. Gone are the days when the doctor knew best and the patient just followed orders. Today, we all have access to more information than ever before, and we can all be *empowered to live happy, healthy, and vibrant lives*. Empowerment drives awareness, responsibility, and accountability for one's health.

CHAPTER 3

Nutrition

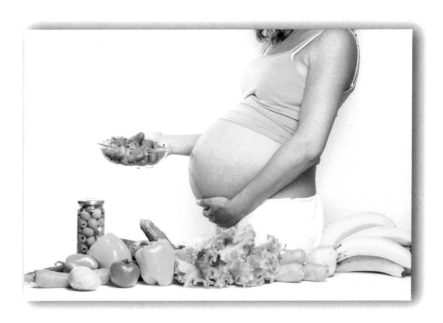

Proper nutrition can require planning and discipline, but so does the wonderful world of parenthood. It is a myth that you need to eat for two. You need to eat for one adult and one growing fetus. The average woman should gain between twenty-five and thirty-five pounds during her pregnancy. Eating for two adults can lead to excessive weight gain and leave you at risk for high blood pressure, gestational diabetes, increased joint pain, heartburn, pelvic floor dysfunction, and potentially, a more challenging delivery. Additionally, the more weight you gain during the pregnancy, the more you have to lose after your pregnancy.

Maintaining adequate levels of the healthy essential fat DHA (fish oil) for you and your growing baby is essential. Low dietary intake of DHA will lead your body to strip it from your brain to help with the development of your baby's brain and nervous system.

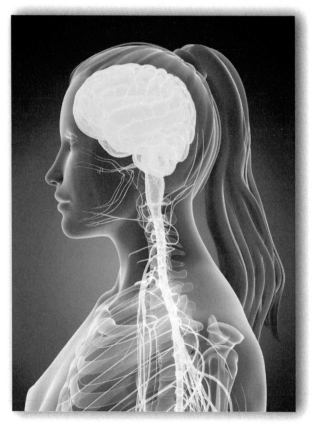

Loss of DHA can cause brain fog during pregnancy or mommy brain after delivery and can lead to very serious postpartum depression. Unfortunately, most food sources that contain DHA also naturally have high levels of contaminants like heavy metals, as in fish, and their consumption must be very limited during pregnancy for fear of toxicity to your unborn baby.

Both during and after pregnancy, it is very important to use a high-quality DHA supplement that has been tested to be free of contaminants. This will help ensure that both you and your baby have ready access to the essential building blocks for the development of the baby's brain and nervous system and will decrease the chance that your developing baby will take them from yours. If your provider does not talk to you about DHA supplementation, then you must be proactive and seek it out yourself.

A healthy nutritional balance will help you maintain energy levels by keeping you properly fueled. Your sense of self and your general attitude may be more positive if you are adequately nourished and hydrated.

Food safety is important for everyone, but it is especially important for you and your unborn baby during pregnancy. You are what you eat, or rather, you are what your mommy eats, drinks, and exposes herself to, is true for your baby during this critical time. Your immune system is suppressed due to hormonal changes, so you must do everything you can to stay as healthy as possible. Eat clean, fresh, organic, healthy foods whenever possible. Make sure to wash your fruits and vegetables and properly cook all meats.

Organic food is grown with very limited or no use of harmful herbicides and pesticides and will not be genetically modified. Grass-fed meat and free-range poultry will have healthier fats in them and will actually have healthy conjugated linoleic acid (CLA) and omega-3 fats. Limit or avoid fish during pregnancy to avoid possible heavy metal exposure. If you do eat fish after your baby is born, make sure it is wild caught and not farm raised, as only the wild caught fish have healthy fats in them.

Eating Healthy

Each meal should contain a combination of healthy, nutrient-dense sources of carbohydrates, protein, and healthy fats. By making nutrition a priority and planning ahead, you will develop a healthy eating habit. Remember, you are going to have a little one watching you very closely in the near future. Your behaviors will form the basis of the habits that your baby will develop. He or she will be a sponge, soaking up everything around him or her, and it all starts in the womb.

Here are some suggestions for what you should be eating and drinking on a daily basis. These are the building blocks for creating a baby inside of you. Just as when building a house (foundation, walls, floors, ceiling, and roof), it takes many different components to create your baby. Your baby needs a balance of high-quality carbohydrates, fats, proteins, vitamins, and minerals.

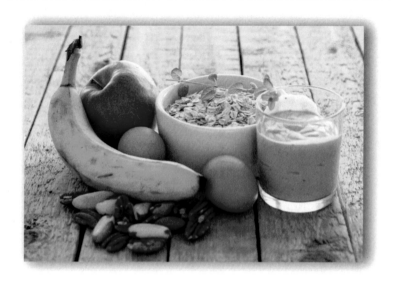

Breakfast

Breakfast is the most important meal of the day for many reasons. Your body has been fasting for eight or more hours. You need to break the fast. Your baby has been taking the nutrition it needs from your body to grow during that time, and you need to replenish your reserves for both you and the baby. Your blood sugar is low, causing your brain to have to work harder to focus. You may get light-headed easily, and if your blood sugar gets too low, you could faint. This is one of the best times for your body to absorb nutrients, so please feed it healthy, high-quality foods.

Here are some high-quality food choices (visit the "Nutrition" page of HemmettHealth.com for more recipes and food choices):

- eggs and fruit
- oatmeal, fruit, and one tablespoon of coconut oil

- Greek yogurt and granola or fruit with one tablespoon of coconut oil
- nut butter on a bagel
- protein shake with fifteen to twenty grams of protein, frozen fruit, coconut oil, and coconut or almond milk (See the "Nutrition" page of HemmettHealth.com for the recipe.)
- homemade protein bar (See the "Nutrition" page of HemmettHealth.com for the recipe.)

Here are some poor-quality food choices:

- only fruit—it is high in sugar without any protein or healthy fats
- sugary cereal—it is almost pure sugar
- only coffee or tea—these beverages have no nutritional value
- toast with margarine—it only provides carbs and un-healthy trans-fatty acids
- no breakfast—your body will continue to starve

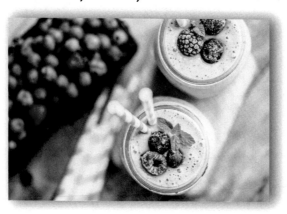

Midmorning Snack

Consistently eating small portions throughout the day will give your body and your baby the consistent supply of building blocks that you both need to flourish. It will also help with or prevent heartburn and reflux.

Here are some examples of healthy, quality snacks:

- homemade protein bar
- organic protein bar
- organic protein shake
- homemade protein shake
- fruit and yogurt
- nuts or seeds and milk
- veggies and nut butter

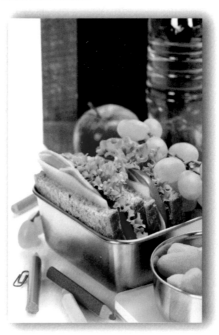

Lunch

Eat a decently sized lunch with a mixture of healthy carbohydrates, protein, and healthy fats. This is a great time for a large, fresh salad with nuts or oil, such as olive, hemp, nut, or seed oil. Or leftovers from dinner the night before is an easy lunch option. A sandwich or wrap with meat and veggies can add variety to lunch.

Don't eat junk food, like chips, pretzels, and sugary foods. These are empty calories and will cause you to gain excessive weight without providing any nutritional value.

Midafternoon Snack

Good options for a midafternoon snack are the same as for a midmorning snack.

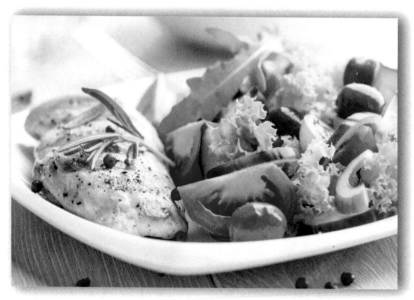

Dinner

Enjoy a healthy balance of carbohydrates, fats, and protein. Try not to eat after seven o'clock. You want to give your body time to digest before bed. This will decrease the chance of reflux. Fresh vegetables are a great source of fiber and essential nutrients. Try to choose a few vegetables so that your plate looks like a colorful rainbow. Different-colored veggies contain different vitamins, so be sure to eat a varied and abundant portion of vegetables. Pair your colorful vegetables with a four- to six-ounce portion of grass-fed or free-range beef, chicken, or turkey for a satisfying, healthy dinner option.

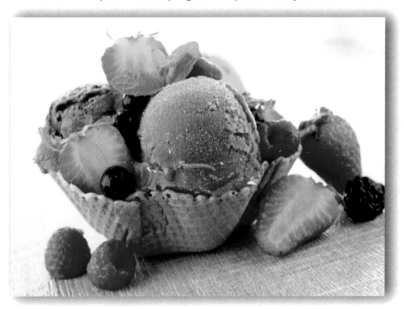

Dessert

It is OK to splurge and have dessert, but portion size is important. Do not eat the whole pint of ice cream! Pay attention to suggested portion sizes. Cravings are common, and it is OK to indulge them, but remember portion size, and remember to try not to eat after seven o'clock or within two hours before bed.

We recommend that you plan ahead and make menus for one-month intervals. This gets you in a routine of healthy eating and lets you plan for shopping and preparation. Weekends are a great time to prepare for the rest of the week. Chop fruit and veggies on Sunday night. Have bread, veggies, and meats ready to go during the work week. We have made a suggested two-week menu and shopping list with some recipes for you on the "Nutrition" page of HemmettHealth.com.

Supplements

Whole-Food Prenatal Vitamin

Here are some important nutrients that should be in your prenatal vitamin:

- 400–800 micrograms (mcg) of folic acid
- 400 IU (international units) of vitamin D
- 200–300 milligrams (mg) of calcium
- 70 mg of vitamin C
- 3 mg of thiamine
- 2 mg of riboflavin
- 20 mg of niacin
- 6 mcg of vitamin B_{12}
- 10 mg of vitamin E

- 15 mg of zinc
- 17 mg of iron
- 150 micrograms of iodine

Folic acid is critical to the development of the baby's brain and nervous system and can prevent many birth defects. One study showed that taking a folic acid supplement for at least a year before conception cut women's chances of delivering early by over 50 percent.

Calcium is critical to bone development in the baby. Taking a supplement with calcium in it can prevent you from losing bone density as the baby takes the calcium it needs from you.

Iodine is crucial for the proper functioning of your thyroid during the pregnancy. A lack of iodine can cause the baby to have mental retardation, stunted growth, and deafness. Iodine deficiency can also lead to miscarriage and stillbirth.

Iron helps the blood in both you and the baby carry essential oxygen.

Some solid prenatal vitamins may cause nausea in some pregnant women. If that happens, you may want a liquid or powdered prenatal vitamin, or you can try taking the solid vitamin at bedtime.

DHA (Docosahexaenoic Acid)

DHA is an omega-3 essential fatty acid that makes up about 20 percent of your brain's cerebral cortex. (*Essential* means that your body cannot make DHA; you have to ingest it in food or supplement form.) DHA plays a very important role in the normal development of the baby in utero. DHA is transferred from you to your developing baby during the last trimester of your pregnancy as the baby's nervous system undergoes a fast growth spurt. Omega-3 fish oils have been shown to increase birth weight and gestational length, support attention and focus in infants and children, support a healthy immune system in infants, support intelligence markers in children, and promote healthy development of the fetal brain, eyes, nervous system, and immune system. There has even been some research showing that children of women who took a supplement with DHA in it during pregnancy and while lactating had higher IQ levels at age four than those who did not.

Besides all the important things DHA does for your baby, it supports your mood and nervous system as well. Taking DHA postnatally can significantly lower your risk of developing postpartum depression.

Your DHA levels will decrease substantially during the pregnancy and will stay low for up to twelve months after delivery unless you take a supplement. Choose a good, clean supplement that provides you with a minimum of 300 mg (preferably 450–900 mg) DHA per serving per day. The label should say that every batch is third-party tested for environmental toxins, including heavy metals, dioxins, and PCBs. Certificates of Analysis should be available upon request. Make sure it is fresh and not oxidized by smelling it. There should only be a faint fishy smell.

DHA is best taken with a meal or food that also has fat in it, so that it is most effectively absorbed. If you burp a fish flavor or get indigestion from the fish oil then try freezing the capsules and taking them with dinner. If that does not work, change brands.

Vitamin D₃

Taking 4,000 IU of vitamin D_3 daily during pregnancy may significantly decrease your risk of preterm birth, gestational diabetes, and infection. Infants with very low levels of vitamin D_3 are at risk of rickets, a disease causing soft bones.

If you or your health care provider are concerned about taking too much vitamin D_3, ask your health care professional to order blood testing to measure your vitamin D_3 levels, and then supplement with D_3 to raise your levels to the high end of the normal range, and take a maintenance dose after that. Usually, most people need 1,000–4,000 IU of vitamin D_3 per day for a maintenance dose.

CHAPTER 4

Prenatal Empowerment Strategies

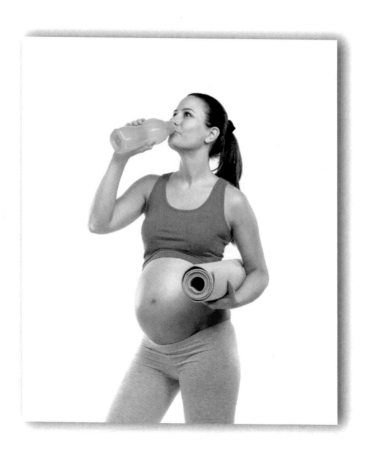

Hydration

Your body needs to increase its blood volume for the growing baby, and additional water will be required. Hydration is key. Carry a water bottle with you everywhere, and drink from it regularly. Try to drink at least sixty-four ounces of water a day. Set a goal of taking five gulps of water every hour. Yes, you will have to go to the restroom a lot, but that is natural. You have an excuse: you are pregnant! If you find that you continue to have bladder challenges after pregnancy, then read our next book on pelvic floor care, and seek treatment for it.

You can mix up your hydration routine by adding a slice of lemon or lime or some maple syrup to your water or by purchasing or making your own carbonated water and adding the above to it.

Make sure the water does not have any artificial sweeteners, flavors, or colors in it. Make sure your water bottle does not contain BPA. A stainless steel or glass water bottle would be the best.

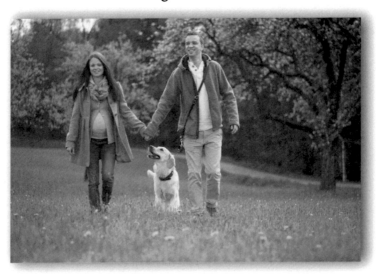

Rest

In general, it is very important to stay as active as possible during your pregnancy. This is why it is so important to take care of yourself, eat right, and try to prevent conditions before they start. Being overly sedentary can lead to high blood pressure, excessive weight gain, and gestational diabetes, or, worst of all, blood clots. Make sure you listen to the recommendations of your prenatal health care team.

Go for a walk in the evenings. Make sure you wear good, supportive walking or running shoes, preferably with a custom-molded orthotic in them. Do not set any records. Keep a pace just fast enough that you start to lose your breath and can no longer only breathe through your nose but must start to breathe through your mouth.

If you are not currently exercising regularly, set a goal to go for a walk for just ten minutes per day. When you return from the walk, perform the daily prenatal exercises and stretches (see chapter 8), and apply ice to any area that you have had challenges with in the past. See how you feel the next day. If you are a little sore but it only lasts for a few hours (up to half a day), then try increasing the time you walk by five minutes, and repeat the daily prenatal exercises and stretches, and icing. Again, see how you do the next day. You can continue doing this up until the point that your soreness lasts the entire next day or the soreness increases in intensity. This is a sign that you have reached your maximum amount of walking.

If you begin to notice that you are having some edema (swelling) in your feet and ankles, then make sure to elevate and ice your feet and ankles for ten to fifteen minutes after you walk and stretch. If you ever notice any one-sided swelling in your legs, especially in the thigh, or calf, then contact your ob-gyn, and let him or her know, as this can be a sign of a more serious condition such as a blood clot.

Mommy-to-Be Empowerment Pack

Prepare yourself with the following items:

- two gel ice packs with covers
- sacroiliac or low-back brace
- high-quality fish oil, prenatal vitamin, and vitamin D$_3$ supplements
- *Prenatal Care* book
- *Postnatal Care* book
- *Pelvic Floor Care* book
- orthotics
- a good pair of walking or running shoes
- two king-size pillows to go between the legs
- physioball
- water bottle

Being prepared will empower you to manage the challenges of pregnancy and parenthood. There will certainly be issues along the way that will require you to make healthy choices for both you and your baby. Taking a little time now to prepare will save you a lot of time and stress later.

CHAPTER 5

The Relaxin Paradox

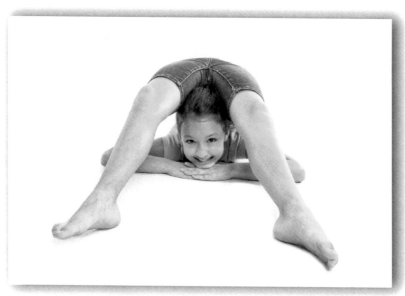

Pregnancy triggers a wide range of changes in a woman's body. The hormone relaxin is produced in both pregnant and nonpregnant females; it rises to a peak within approximately fourteen days of ovulation and then declines in the absence of pregnancy. During the first trimester of pregnancy, levels rise. Relaxin reaches its peak during the fourteen weeks of the first trimester and at delivery.

Relaxin acts to loosen ligaments and plays an essential role in allowing the pelvic canal to open as the baby descends during the birthing process. The challenge is that this hormone does not just target the ligaments of the joints of the pelvis but acts globally to loosen all the body's ligaments, including the joints of the lower back, hips, knees, ankles, and feet. All the ligaments attached to the twenty-six bones of the feet loosen. Since relaxin levels elevate early in the pregnancy, these changes can occur for months, and combined with increased weight gain, increased fluid retention, and changes in the center of gravity of the pelvis, they can create significant challenges for the lower back, hips, knees, ankles, and feet.

Biomechanical changes to the feet and changes in gait that are triggered by the increased relaxin production can become permanent and last after birth. This is why it is very important to approach your pregnancy as proactively as possible and not just accept the fact that because your mom or aunt or friend had problems, you are destined to have them as well. Many challenges are common but not normal.

We recommend that every pregnant woman wear a custom orthotic. Visit HemmettHealth.com to read about the companies we feel are the best. If you cannot find a provider to fit you for orthotics, or if there is a financial barrier, then at least use a noncustomized orthotic. Again, you can find recommendations on our website. We will update these products as we encounter new high-quality products.

Always wear good, supportive shoes, like walking or running shoes, with your orthotics in them. Yes, this includes in the house. We will repeat—always wear good, supportive shoes, like walking or running shoes, with your orthotics, even in the house. Never wear flip-flops or go barefoot unless you are performing your foot-strengthening exercises. You may try using the X Brace elastic foot brace to support your arch during activities like yoga if you are not allowed to wear shoes, but we still feel that shoes with orthotics are the best. Dress shoes should always be worn with your orthotics, as they are notoriously unsupportive.

CHAPTER 6

Warnings

Your body changes at such a rapid rate during pregnancy that it may be a challenge to know what symptoms may be a sign of a more serious issue. A general rule of thumb is if in doubt, call your health care provider and ask.

Call your medical birthing health care provider right away if you experience any of the following:

- unusual or severe cramping or abdominal pain
- noticeable changes in your baby's movement after twenty-eight weeks' gestation (if you don't count ten movements within two hours)
- difficulty breathing or shortness of breath that seems to be getting worse
- signs of premature labor, including the following:
    - regular tightening or pain in the lower abdomen or back
    - any bleeding in the second or third trimester
    - a fluid leak

- severe pressure in the pelvis or vagina (pressure is normal in the second and third trimesters)

Also call your health care provider if you have any of the following conditions during pregnancy:

- a fever over one hundred degrees Fahrenheit
- severe or persistent vomiting
- severe diarrhea
- fainting spells or dizziness
- pain, burning, or trouble urinating
- unusual vaginal discharge
- vaginal bleeding
- swelling in your hands, fingers, or face
- blurred vision or spots before your eyes
- sore, cracked, or bleeding nipples
- severe headaches
- blurred vision
- pain or cramping in your arms, legs, or chest

The vast majority of symptoms that you will experience are not a sign of a very serious issue. Empowering yourself through open communication with all of your health care providers will give you the peace of mind to enjoy your pregnancy and know what is, and what is not, a serious concern that needs to be dealt with immediately.

CHAPTER 7

Common Prenatal Orthopedic
Conditions, and What to Do about Them

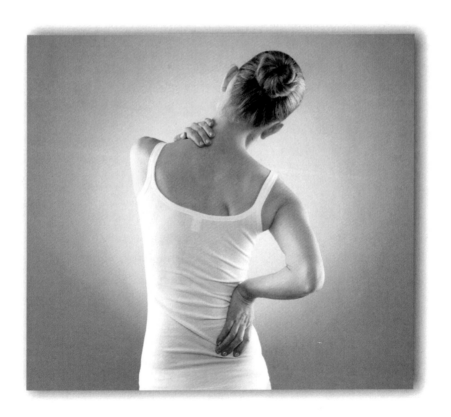

The Aches and Pains of Pregnancy

Pregnancy causes your body to transform at a rate far faster than during any other normal adult process. Hormones fluctuate, and your center of gravity changes over a relatively short period of time, and together, these changes alter your gait. You gain weight, while at the same time, your ligaments become overly stretchy and provide less stability to your joints. Muscles easily get overworked, and pain can develop. Pregnancy is the great magnifying glass. It will magnify any little imbalance that you have in your neuro-musculoskeletal system (nerves, muscles, joints, ligaments, tendons, and fascia).

We would like to warn you: recently, a research study showed that taking over-the-counter acetaminophen for a prolonged period of time during pregnancy was associated with increased risk for ADHD-like behaviors in the child. This was most common when acetaminophen was taken during the second and third trimesters. We recommend trying to treat your pain in a safe, conservative manner, and if you feel you must take acetaminophen, then discuss it first with your birthing professional, and limit your intake as much as possible.[1]

Changes in Your Core

The core is composed of the musculature of the diaphragm, deep abdominals, and pelvic floor. A strong, conditioned core is essential to support and control the individual spinal and pelvic

---

1 Stergiakouli,2016

joints and provide a solid, neutral upper foundation for the hips and legs. It also protects the discs and nerves of the back and allows them to function in a neutral position.

A weak core going into pregnancy, changes in the center of gravity of your pelvis during pregnancy, increased ligamentous laxity (looseness) in the back, pelvis, hips, and feet, as well as the baby descending and pushing the abdomen outward all contribute toward making it increasingly difficult to keep a strong core throughout the pregnancy. The sooner you get started strengthening and conditioning the core, the better. However, it is never too late to do some breathing exercises, Kegel-type pelvic floor contractures, or mild seated pelvic-tilting exercises on a physioball (see "Daily Prenatal Exercises and Stretches").

Unfortunately, a word of caution is needed here. Most core exercise programs that we have seen our patients demonstrate are not actually strengthening the core and are in fact reinforcing overactive hip flexors and underactivating the deep abdominals. In addition, through our work with pelvic floor therapy, our female providers have found that most women (even those who have done pelvic floor therapy) have no idea how to contract all or some of their pelvic floor muscles. See our book on pelvic floor care for more details on that.

The traditional swayback—or hyperlordosis—often seen in pregnancy is the result of underuse of the core. It is important to think about lifting the baby up and back and not letting it pull the pelvis forward and down. This poor posture will be reinforced by improper core exercise techniques, so be careful. In general, if an exercise is painful to do, you should not be doing it. If you feel worse immediately after doing the exercise or the next day, then you should seek help from a trained professional or a different trained professional.

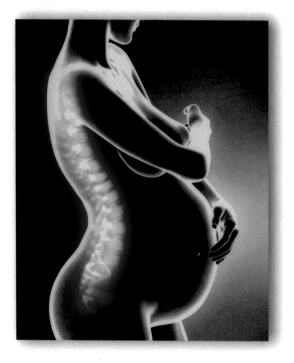

It is very common for the hip flexors to become overactive and shortened as the pelvis tilts forward. These are very strong muscles that originate at the low-back joints and discs and come forward and down to the hips. The hip flexors will put a lot of pressure on the joints and discs of the lower back as well as on the hips themselves.

Every pregnant woman, regardless of whether she is having problems or not, should stretch her hip flexors every night for thirty seconds three times on each side. While you are doing this, you should lift the baby up and back with your lower abdominal muscles. It would be even better for you to do the daily prenatal exercises and stretches.

Preparation for Your Recovery

Preparation is key. Working on your core and other areas during pregnancy sets the stage for your recovery postnatally. By preparing your body for pregnancy, you can give yourself the best possible chance to mitigate the potential for significant debilitating pain during your pregnancy and to reclaim your body after pregnancy. You've already started preparing by reading this book.

We highly recommend planning and preparing for your postnatal recovery as soon as possible. It is inevitable that your body will become deconditioned and change, no matter what you do, so you might as well plan for it and become empowered to give yourself the best possible chance to have a happy, healthy, and vibrant pregnancy and postnatal recovery. We are writing a postnatal care book and a pelvic floor care book to help empower you to regain your body and live well after the delivery.

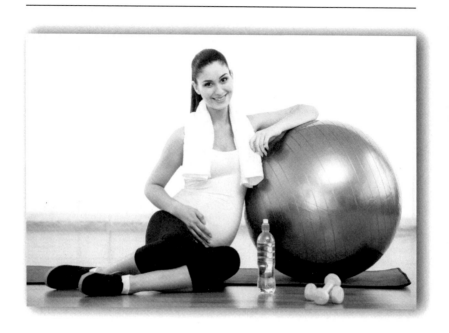

Prehab Wellness Program

Prehab is a supervised prenatal strength and conditioning program that we have developed in our clinics to help women reach their potential fitness levels during the prenatal process. It combines in-office, professionally monitored therapy and home-based exercises. It is designed to adapt to your changing body and prepare it for delivery and postnatal recovery.

General Care Guidelines

Perform the prescribed exercises three times per day, with the last time being before bed. Use ice after you stretch and before bed if that is part of the protocol. If the exercises become painful to do, or if your discomfort does not improve after two weeks of self-care, ask a qualified medical provider for help.

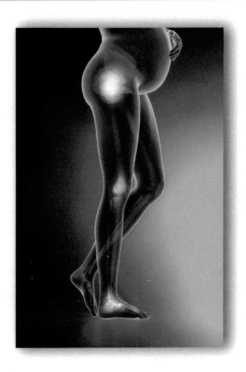

Condition One: Hip and/or Leg Pain (Piriformis Syndrome)

Piriformis syndrome is a condition in which the piriformis muscle, located in the buttock region, spasms and causes localized buttock pain. The piriformis muscle can also irritate the nearby sciatic nerve and cause pain, numbness, and tingling along the back of the leg and into the foot (sciatic pain) or irritate the nearby sacroiliac joint, causing sacroiliac syndrome (see condition three).

The piriformis muscle starts at the lower spine (sacrum) and connects to the upper surface of each femur (thighbone). The piriformis assists in rotating the hip and turning the leg and foot outward. It runs diagonally, with the sciatic nerve running vertically directly beneath it (although in some people, the nerve can run through the muscle).

The two most common dysfunctions leading to spasm of the piriformis muscle that can happen either separately or together are

- hyperpronation of the feet, allowing internal rotation of the femur and causing the piriformis muscle to contract in response, and
- too much anterior tilting of the pelvis (sacral portion) and the resulting change in force on the muscle.

Home- and office-based therapy should be focused on reestablishing as close to neutral foot and pelvic positioning as possible. This is done by reestablishing normal movement of the associated muscles and joints of the lower back, sacroiliac, feet, and hip regions.

Here are some home-care strategies:

1. Self- and partner stretches—1, 2, 3, 8, 10, 11, 14, 17, 18, 22, and 23
2. Partner massage for the following muscles—piriformis, glutes, hamstrings, adductors, and quadriceps
3. Orthotics and proper footwear
4. Proper sleep, sitting, and driving positions

Office care:

1. Soft-tissue techniques—active release, graston, hold-relax post neuromuscular facilitation (PNF), and massage for piriformis, glutes, hamstrings, adductors, quadriceps, and hip flexors
2. Chiropractic joint manipulation for the lower back, sacroiliac, and hips
3. Rehabilitative strengthening exercises to support the feet and core
4. Custom-molded biomechanical orthotics

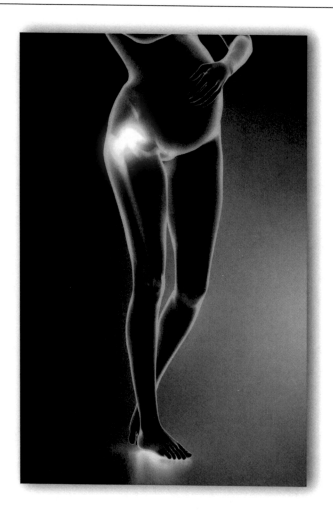

Condition Two: Hip Pain (Bursitis)

Bursitis is inflammation of the fluid-filled sac (bursa) that provides padding between muscles or a muscle and bone. There are two major bursas in the hip that typically become irritated and inflamed. One bursa, called the greater trochanter, covers the bony point of the hip bone. Inflammation of this bursa is called trochanteric bursitis. As your pelvis expands and your center of gravity changes, your hips will be progressively challenged. Any type of dysfunction in the legs, feet, or pelvis can cause the musculature of the hips to get overworked and put too much pressure on your bursa. The musculature will rub on the bursa and cause it to swell and become inflamed and painful. You must correct the abnormal mechanics of the legs and pelvis that cause the dysfunction of the hip musculature.

The two most common dysfunctions that can happen either separately or together are

- hyperpronation of the feet, allowing internal rotation of the femur, and
- too much anterior tilting of the pelvis.

Home and in-office therapy should be focused on reestablishing as close to neutral foot and pelvic positioning as possible. This is done by reestablishing normal movement of the associated muscles and joints of the lower back, sacroiliac, feet, and hip regions.

Here are some home-care strategies:

1. Icing the hip
2. Self- and partner stretches—1, 2, 3, 8, 10, 11, 14, 17, 18, 22, and 23
3. Partner massage for the following muscles—piriformis, glutes, hamstrings, adductors, quadriceps, and hip flexors
4. Orthotics and proper footwear

5. Sleeping with two pillows between the legs and proper sitting and driving positions
6. Seated physioball posterior pelvic tilt (PPT) exercise

Here are some effective in-office care therapies:

1. Soft-tissue therapy—active release, graston, hold-relax post neuromuscular facilitation (PNF), and massage for piriformis, glutes, hamstrings, adductors, quadriceps, and hip flexors
2. Chiropractic joint manipulation—sacroiliac and hip
3. Rehabilitative strengthening exercises for the feet and core
4. Custom-molded biomechanical orthotics

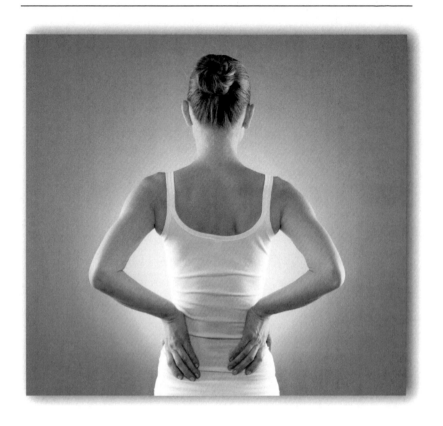

Condition Three: Low-Back and Upper Leg Pain (Sacroiliac Syndrome)

Dysfunction in the sacroiliac joint, or SI joint, is thought to cause low-back and upper leg pain. The leg pain can be particularly difficult and may feel similar to sciatica or pain caused by a lumbar disc herniation. This is often mistaken for, or called, hip pain.

The two most common dysfunctions leading to sacroiliac syndrome that can happen either separately or together are

- hyperpronation of the feet, allowing internal rotation of the femur, and
- too much anterior tilting of the pelvis.

Home and in-office therapy should be focused on reestablishing foot and pelvic positioning as close to neutral as possible. This is done by reestablishing normal movement of the associated muscles and joints of the lower back, sacroiliac, feet, and hip regions.

Here are some home-care strategies:

1. Icing the sacroiliac joint
2. Self- and partner stretches—1, 2, 3, 8, 10, 11, 13, 14, 17, 18, 22, 23, and 24
3. Partner massage for the following muscles—piriformis, glutes, hamstrings, adductors, quadriceps, hip flexors, and Spinal Erectors (lower back)
4. Orthotics and proper footwear
5. Sleeping with two pillows between the legs and proper sitting and driving positions
6. Intermittent use of a sacroiliac belt
7. Rehabilitative strengthening exercises—cat and camel and seated physioball posterior pelvic tilt

Here are some effective in-office care therapies:

1. Soft-tissue therapy—active release, graston, hold-relax post neuromuscular facilitation (PNF), and massage for

piriformis, glutes, hamstrings, adductors, quadriceps, and hip flexors
2. Chiropractic joint manipulation—sacroiliac and hip
3. Rehabilitative strengthening exercises for the feet and core
4. Custom-molded biomechanical orthotics

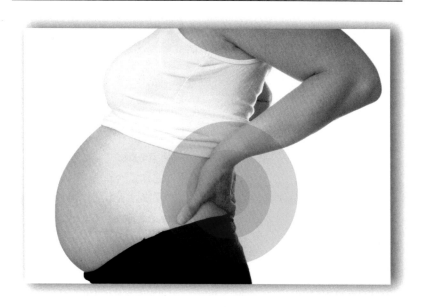

Condition Four: Low-Back Pain

Unfortunately, low-back pain during pregnancy is very common, but it is not normal. As the baby grows, your center of gravity changes, and relaxin production increases; it is common for the pelvis to tilt forward excessively, causing pressure on the joints and discs of the lower back. The cumulative effects of improper sitting posture, poor work habits, incorrect lifting, lack of proper exercise, and other lifestyle-related factors are magnified by the effects of pregnancy. All of these factors cause repetitive, low-level stress on the spinal joints and associated musculature and eventually cause pain. When this occurs, the surrounding back muscles go into spasm to protect the stressed or injured tissues of the back.

The two most common dysfunctions that can happen either separately or together are

- hyperpronation of the feet, allowing internal rotation of the femur, and
- too much anterior tilting of the pelvis.

Home and in-office therapy should be focused on reestablishing foot and pelvic positioning as close to neutral as possible. This is done by reestablishing normal movement of the associated muscles and joints of the lower back, sacroiliac, feet, and hip regions.

Symptoms of lower back pain include the following:

- pain, tenderness, and stiffness in the back or between the shoulder blades
- pain that radiates into the buttocks or to the knee
- difficulty standing straight or in one position for prolonged periods of time
- weakness or leg fatigue when walking
- discomfort while sitting

Here are some home-care strategies:

1. Icing of low back
2. Self- and partner stretches—1, 2, 3, 8, 10, 11, 13, 14, 17, 18, 22, 23, and 24

3. Partner massage for the following muscles—piriformis, glutes, hamstrings, adductors, quadriceps, hip flexors, and spinal erectors (lower back)
4. Orthotics and proper footwear
5. Sleeping with two pillows between the legs and proper sitting and driving positions
6. Intermittent use of a sacroiliac belt
7. Rehabilitative strengthening exercises—cat and camel, and seated physioball posterior pelvic tilt

Here are some effective in-office care therapies:

1. Soft-tissue therapy—active release, graston, hold-relax post neuromuscular facilitation (PNF), and massage for piriformis, glutes, hamstrings, adductors, quadriceps, and hip flexors
2. Chiropractic joint manipulation for the middle back and lower back, and sacroiliac regions
3. Rehabilitative strengthening exercises for the feet and core
4. Custom-molded biomechanical orthotics

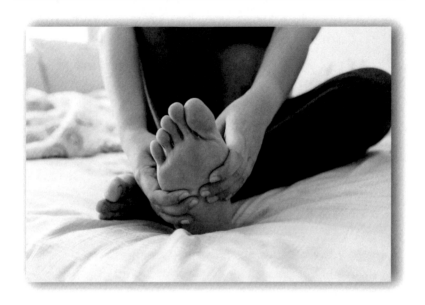

Condition Five: Foot Pain

Foot pain is one of the most commonly overlooked complaints during pregnancy. Two primary changes occur in the foot. The foot volume increases due to edema (swelling), and the foot grows because the ligaments that support the twenty-six bones of the feet loosen.

The surge in the hormone relaxin early in pregnancy, combined with weight gain, edema, and the shift in the center of gravity of the pelvis, causes increased stress on the joints and muscles of the hips, legs, and feet. The result is that the joints of the feet become overloaded and the arches drop, which causes the foot to elongate and puts excessive stress on the plantar fascia ligament on the bottom of the foot, which can result in pain and inflammation in the heel, arch, and ball of the foot. It can also cause existing foot conditions such as calluses, corns, and cracked heels to become painful. This hyperpronation causes even more stress on the feet, knees, hips, and back and can cause you to grow a shoe size and develop the characteristic pregnancy waddle.

It is important to treat hyperpronation for pain relief but also to prevent development of other foot conditions such as plantar fasciitis (heel and mid foot pain), heel spurs, metatarsalgia (pain around the ball of the foot), post-tibialis tendonitis (ankle and shin pain), and bunions. Some research even suggests that the changes in gait during pregnancy related to hyperpronation and elongation of the foot may become permanent, so do not wait until you develop pain to support your feet.

Unfortunately, pain in the hips, knees, and feet during pregnancy is often considered to be normal and is dismissed with the assumption that it will just go away on its own after birth.

Here are some home-care strategies:

1. Icing and elevating the feet
2. Wearing tightly laced, supportive running or walking shoes, and avoiding heels and flip-flops (Put your shoes on first thing in the morning when you have the least swelling.)
3. Self- and partner stretches—1, 2, 3, 8, 9, 11, 17, 18, and 22
4. Partner massage for the following muscles—piriformis, glutes, hamstrings, adductors, calves, and feet
5. Orthotics—the hyperpronation associated with pregnancy is best treated with a truly custom, biomechanically correct foot orthotic. Raising the arch will shorten

it back to its neutral length. The orthotic may also help your knee, hip, and low-back pain. A custom orthotic that your practitioner can adjust is best so that he or she can raise and lower it, if needed, during the pregnancy. The earlier you intervene, the better in order to give yourself the best chance to benefit from the orthotics and to avoid other conditions like plantar fasciitis (heel and mid foot pain), bunions, and metatarsalgia (pain around the ball of the foot).

6. Rehabilitative exercises—toe curls to strengthen the muscles of the foot. They complement the passive support to the ligaments offered by the custom orthotics.

Here are some effective in-office care therapies:

1. Soft-tissue therapies—active release, graston, massage, and hold-relax post neuromuscular facilitation (PNF) for piriformis, glutes, hamstrings, adductors, quadriceps, hip flexors, calves, and intrinsic foot muscles
2. Chiropractic joint manipulation for the feet
3. Rehabilitative strengthening exercises for the feet
4. Custom-molded biomechanical orthotics

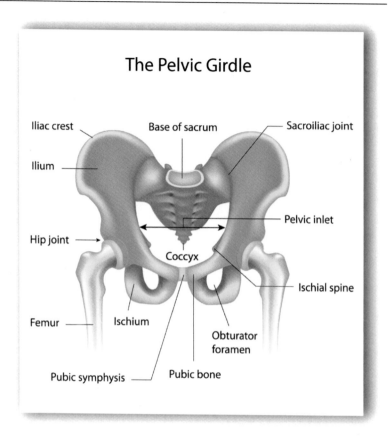

The Pelvic Girdle

Iliac crest

Base of sacrum

Sacroiliac joint

Ilium

Hip joint

Pelvic inlet

Coccyx

Ischial spine

Femur

Ischium

Obturator foramen

Pubic symphysis

Pubic bone

Condition Six: Pubic Pain

The pubic symphysis (PS) joint and the two sacroiliac joints are the three joints that compromise the pelvic ring where the baby must descend through the birth canal. The pubic symphysis needs to increase in width, and anything that either inhibits this or leads to instability at this area can trigger pain here. Excessive anterior pelvic tilting can lead to too much tension on the pyramidalis muscle, leading to pain at the pubic symphysis. You may have pain on the inside of your legs. It may be painful to sleep on your side at night. There may be grinding or popping in the area. Getting up at night to go to the bathroom may be very painful. Most activities requiring a single-leg stance, such as climbing stairs, will cause pain and become very challenging. Lack of motion in the sacroiliac joints may lead to excessive movement at the PS and cause pain.

Here are some home-care strategies:

1. Icing the pubic symphysis
2. Self- and partner stretches—1, 2, 3, 8, 10, 11, 14, 17, 18, 22, and 23
3. Partner massage for the following muscles—piriformis, glutes, hamstrings, adductors, and quadriceps
4. Orthotics and proper footwear
5. Sleeping with two pillows between the legs and proper sitting and driving positions
6. Intermittent use of a sacroiliac belt

Here are some effective in-office care therapies:

1. Soft-tissue therapies—active release, hold-relax post neuromuscular facilitation (PNF), graston, and massage for piriformis, glutes, hamstrings, adductors, quadriceps, and pyramidalis
2. Chiropractic joint manipulation for the pubic symphysis, sacroiliac, and hips
3. Rehabilitative exercises for the core
4. Custom-molded biomechanical orthotics

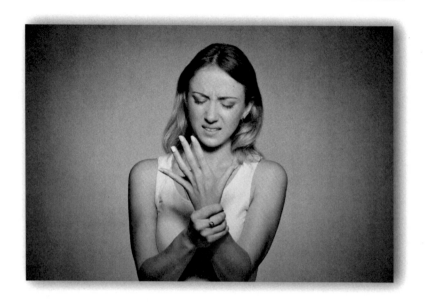

Condition Seven: Hand Numbness and Tingling (Carpal Tunnel Syndrome and Thoracic Outlet Syndrome)

Numbness and tingling in the hands can be caused by the systemic increase in fluid and blood volume associated with pregnancy. Women who use their hands repetitively or for prolonged periods of time (such as for typing, writing, carrying children, cutting hair, or preparing food) or who sleep with their arms, hands, and wrists in poor positions are at increased risk of developing numbness and tingling in the hands during pregnancy; this is called carpal tunnel syndrome. Women with poor posture (such as when the head is held forward and not centered at the top of the spine) are also at increased risk for developing numbness and tingling in the hands during pregnancy; this is called thoracic outlet syndrome.

The carpal tunnel in the wrist is a space that has a fixed volume because the retinaculum, or bracelet, of ligaments that stabilizes the wrist is not flexible. As the fluid volume increases in the tunnel, it will put pressure on the nerves and other structures in the tunnel. When these nerves become squeezed by this pressure, numbness and tingling sensations can result and can ultimately lead to weakness in the hands as well. Use of the hands may make this worse. The symptoms may come and go, be constant, or be related to use or position, such as first thing in the morning after sleeping in a poor position.

The thoracic outlet is an area in the front and sides of the neck where your scalene muscles originate in your neck and attach to your ribs. These muscles pass over the top of the nerves and blood vessels that go from your neck to your arms and hands. When you have poor posture during the day or even a poor sleeping posture at night, your scalene muscles tighten up and can put pressure on the nerves and blood vessels, which can cause numbness and tingling down the arms and hands and even weakness in the arms and hands.

Here are some home-care strategies:

1. Icing the hands and wrists
2. Self- and partner stretches—4, 5, 7, 15, 16, 19, and 21
3. Partner massage for levator scapula, upper trapezius, pectoralis, and forearm flexors
4. Elevating the hands and arms in the evening

5. Sleeping with wrists and elbows straight, and possibly with a carpal tunnel wrist brace, and proper sitting and driving positions

Here are some effective in-office care therapies:

1. Soft-tissue therapies—active release, graston, hold-relax post neuromuscular facilitation (PNF), and massage for forearm flexors, transverse carpal ligaments, intrinsic hand muscles, and scalene muscles.
2. Chiropractic joint manipulation for the wrists and neck
3. Rehabilitative exercises for the neck and hands
4. Ergonomic and posture training for daily activities and sleep

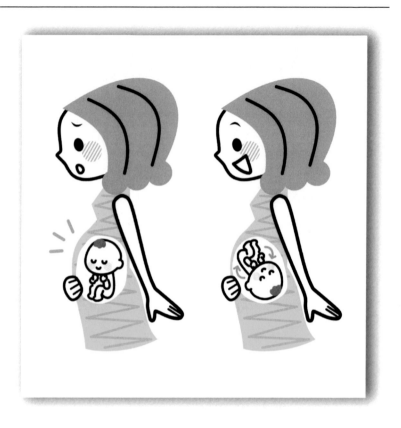

Condition Eight: Breech Presentation

A breech presentation occurs in pregnancy when the baby is head up in the uterus instead of being head down and prepared for delivery. In the vast majority of cases where the baby is in a breech position, a C-section is required. There are some musculoskeletal components of the uterine ligaments and pelvis that can become tight and restricted during pregnancy, which may be related to the malposition of the baby.

Hemmett Health providers have developed a safe, noninvasive therapy to help restore sacroiliac, hip, and pubic symphysis range of motion and to decrease muscle tension to help relax the pelvis. The technique gently releases tension within the soft tissues to allow the baby to move more easily in utero. The doctors will assess the movement of your sacroiliac joints and palpate the tone of your round ligament on the abdomen. Following proper diagnosis, they will perform gentle mobilization and soft-tissue release techniques to free restrictions in the affected structures. There is no direct palpation of the baby! This technique focuses on the optimal movement within your pelvic structures to allow for more freedom of movement within your uterus and thus provide more room for your baby to turn. This is a safe, gentle, and conservative approach to allow your baby to move into an optimal head-down position.

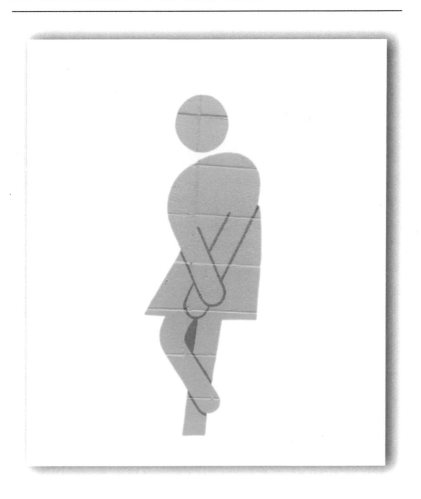

Condition Nine: Postnatal Urinary Incontinence
Research suggests that learning and performing pelvic floor strengthening exercises before conception and during pregnancy may decrease the chances of developing permanent urinary incontinence. It is extremely common to experience and develop urinary incontinence (leakage or peeing your pants) after childbirth (or C-section). This condition can become a problematic

social barrier for physical activity and results in real feelings of isolation and desperation. Thankfully, there is a conservative, effective, and relatively quick permanent solution.[23]

Work with your health care professional to develop a prenatal pelvic floor strengthening program. In our next two books, *Postnatal Care* and *Pelvic Floor Care*, we will discuss how to effectively treat postnatal urinary incontinence if it does occur. Healthy, strong and flexible, pelvic floor muscles are the key to combatting postnatal urinary incontinence. Although common, postnatal urinary incontinence is not normal, and does not have to be accepted.

2 Haddow,2005
3 Morkved,2014

CHAPTER 8

Home-Care Strategies

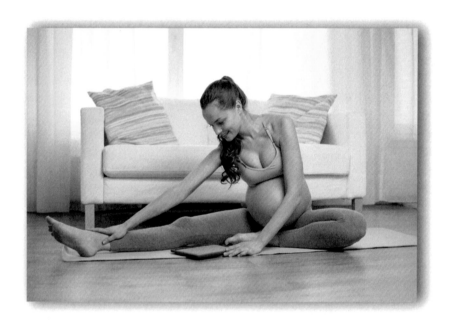

Actively participating in your pregnancy is crucial to enjoying a healthy pregnancy. Active participation will give you some control over your body and how you feel, both mentally and physically. Do not ignore your body's warning signs of pain and dysfunction, and do no rely on a health care provider to fix you. Actively participate with your health care provider in order to achieve the best possible outcomes.

Self-Care Guidelines

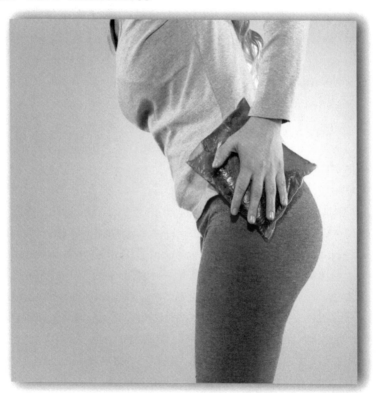

Guidelines for Icing

The goal of icing is to limit inflammation and pain and therefore decrease the amount of protective muscle spasm that will take place.

DR. VICKI HEMMETT & DR. ERIK HEMMETT

Icing works best on joints that are sore, painful, and inflamed. Place a damp towel on the area to be iced, and then apply the ice pack or plastic bag containing ice cubes over the area. Leave the ice in place for twenty minutes, and then take it off for thirty minutes, and then you may repeat. If the icing becomes painful, then use a thicker damp towel. Make sure not to apply the ice directly to unprotected skin. The primary joints that need icing are the lumbar (low-back) facet, both sacroiliacs, hips, pubic symphysis, and feet. Icing is best done while standing or lying down on your side. When standing, you can simply secure the towel and ice in place with your sacroiliac belt or low-back belt and continue doing what you need to.

Guidelines for Stretching
Always warm up before stretching. Do not go from being seden-tary (sitting, lying down, or sleeping) right to stretching. Make sure to walk around and warm up for at least thirty minutes first. Use gentle tension with no bouncing. There should be no sharp pain. Stretching may cause short-term soreness in the area for up to twenty-four hours, but it should not last longer than that. If it does, try stretching less aggressively, and make sure to let your health care team know. The primary muscles that need to be stretched during pregnancy are the psoas, piriformis, glutes, adductors, and gastroc and soleus in the calf.

Guidelines for Partner Massage and Stretching
Soft-tissue work may be slightly painful and cause soreness for up to twenty-four hours afterward. The goal is not to beat up

the tissue but to regularly, gently coax it into relaxing. Having your partner help you with stretches or massage gives him or her a role to help you and helps develop a bond of understanding about the changes your body is going through. It is better for your partner to start lightly and then over time, gradually increase the pressure. You can always do more next time, but you cannot take back what you have already done.

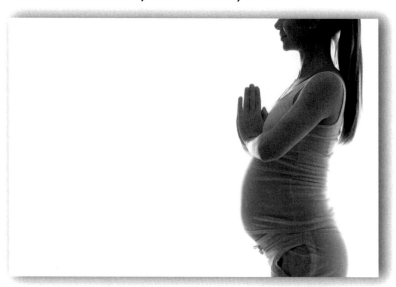

Guidelines for Ergonomics and Posture
As you progress through the pregnancy, it is very common for your shoulders and head to round forward, your pelvis to tilt forward, your hips to rotate inward, and the arches in your feet to drop. This all happens as a result of relaxin production and subsequent ligamentous laxity, as well as because of weight gain and the shift in your center of gravity. It is important to try to maintain neutral

joint positions by keeping the chin and shoulders back and down, the pelvis in a neutral position by lifting the baby up and back, and the feet supported. We recommend using orthotics at all times in addition to doing strengthening exercises for the intrinsic muscles of the feet. The less you allow the joints in your feet to deform, the less likely they will be to cause you problems during and after the pregnancy. A high, semirigid custom orthotic is the best, but if that is not an option, a noncustom orthotic that is as rigid and high as possible is second best. At a minimum, use a good walking or running shoe as much as possible, and avoid high heels and narrow, unsupportive pumps. Use a supportive shoe indoors, if possible. If you already practice yoga or take it up during pregnancy, make sure to focus on maintaining a high arch in your feet while standing at all times in addition to using an x-brace to help open up the hips and keep them in a neutral position. In some cases when you have pain, you should use a supportive shoe with an orthotic during yoga.

Something done once for a short period of time, whether it is good or bad, will not have a significant effect on you (unless it is a big trauma). However, something like posture and ergonomics that you do repetitively or for long periods on a regular basis will have a huge impact on you over time. So, let's get started!

Perform stretching aggressively enough to feel tension and not pain. Do not bounce. A gentle stretch done frequently is more effective than an aggressive stretch done once weekly. No exercises should increase sharp pain or cause shooting pain into the extremities. Sometimes, a temporary increase in numbness and tingling while stretching is normal, but be sure to make your provider aware.

The great news is that you will have the ability to make some long-term changes that will have a significant positive effect on your body. The bad news is that by default, your body will degenerate over time, no matter what you do or do not do. However, the speed at which it degenerates is mostly impacted by your daily habits.

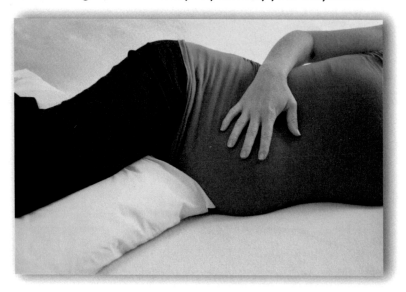

Guidelines for Sleeping

Use two pillows stacked together between your knees and feet when you sleep on your side, and keep your knees parallel and legs straight. Do not bend your knees up to your chest. Bending them up to the chest will cause your psoas (hip flexor) muscles to shorten and put pressure on your lower back. Tighten your lower abdominal muscles to lift the baby up and back before you roll over or try to get out of bed. Keep the pillows between your legs when you roll over in bed.

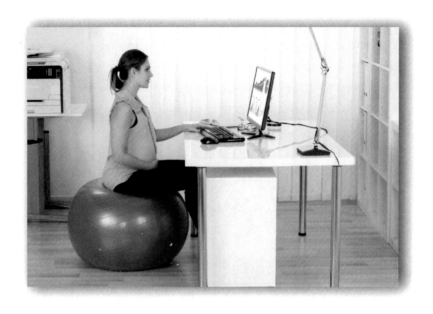

Guidelines for Sitting

Every thirty minutes, take a break from sitting to stand or stretch. Keep your hips higher than your knees. Do not sit cross-legged as this will cause your piriformis muscles to shorten. Keep your hips, knees, and feet facing straight ahead. Keep your elbows by your sides; do not reach forward for your keyboard or mouse. Stay close enough to your desk to keep your elbows by your side. Keep your elbows higher than your wrists, and keep your shoulders and head back. When you have the opportunity, elevate your feet with ice on them for twenty minutes to help with swelling but then return to the neutral sitting position.

Guidelines for Driving

Keep your hips higher than your knees. Keep your hips, knees, and feet facing straight ahead. Do not rotate either foot outward. Keep your elbows by your side. Use an underhand grip on the steering wheel, with your hands at eight and four o'clock to avoid reaching your arms forward and slouching your head and shoulders.

Routine Daily Prenatal Exercises

#1: 3 sets 10 reps each

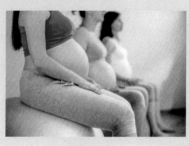

#2: Hold each position 15 to 30

Seconds repeat 2 to 4 times

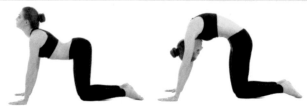

#3: Repeat 5 to 10 times each side

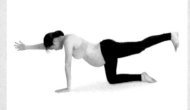

#4: Brisk 15 minute walk

#5: Stretches # 1,2,3,4,5,7,8,9,10,11,14,15,16

#6: Ice sore areas

Daily Prenatal Exercises and Stretches

It is important that you do not wait for pain to start and that you be proactive. Perform these exercises every evening at dinnertime or before bed when you are not having pain. An ounce of prevention can sometimes be stronger than a pound of cure.

Exercise One: Physioball Seated Posterior Pelvic Tilt

Inflate your physioball to the height at which your hips are slightly higher than your knees when you sit on it. Most women will need a sixty-five centimeter ball. Sit on the ball. You can find center by gently bouncing up and down until you can almost lift your legs off the ground and be balanced. Stop bouncing. Begin the exercise by tightening your lower abdominal muscles and using the muscles to lift your baby up and back. This will naturally tuck your tailbone underneath you. Make sure to keep your torso upright and your head and shoulders back and down. Do not slouch. The ball should not move much. Relax, and return to the starting positon. You can exhale as you tighten your abdominals and inhale as you return to the starting position. You can also try to tighten your pelvic floor muscles at the same time as you tighten your lower abdominals. This should be a very comfortable exercise and should not cause any pain. Keep your hips higher than your knees and your knees and feet straight ahead and hip width apart. As you get into the late stages of your third trimester, you may need to spread your knees apart more. Hold the contracture for a couple of seconds, and then relax.

Repeat this ten times, and do three sets of ten total. You can also sit and do gentle clockwise and counterclockwise circles on the ball.

See picture of daily prenatal exercise 1.

Exercise Two: Cat and Camel

Get down on your hands and knees on the floor. Relax your head, and allow it to droop. Round your back up toward the ceiling until you feel a nice stretch in your upper, middle, and lower back. Hold this stretch for as long as it feels comfortable (about fifteen to thirty seconds). Return to the starting position with a flat back. Then, let your back sway by pressing your stomach toward the floor. Lift your buttocks toward the ceiling. Hold this position for fifteen to thirty seconds. Repeat two to four times.

See picture of daily prenatal exercise 2.

Exercise Three: Quadruped

Position yourself on your hands and knees on an exercise mat or a carpeted floor. Your hands should be roughly shoulder width apart, and your knees and feet should be roughly hip width apart. Contract your abdominal muscles, and maintain a flat back throughout the movement. Extend one leg at the knee and hip out behind you while simultaneously extending the opposite arm in front of you. Both the leg and arm should be straight and parallel to the floor. Return to the start positon and repeat for the opposite arm and leg. This is one repetition. Do this five to ten times.

Make sure to keep your torso (the abdominals and back) tight during the entire exercise.

See picture of daily prenatal exercise 3.

Exercise Four: Brisk Fifteen-Minute Walk

Keep up a pace that allows you to breathe through your nose. Try to stay on a flat surface. Wear supportive walking or running sneakers, preferably with arch supports in them.

Exercise Five: Stretches

See prenatal self-stretches 1, 2, 3, 4, 5, 7, 8, 9, 10, 11, 14, 15, and 16.

Exercise Six: Ice

Ice any areas that are sore Refer to the "Guidelines for Icing" section.

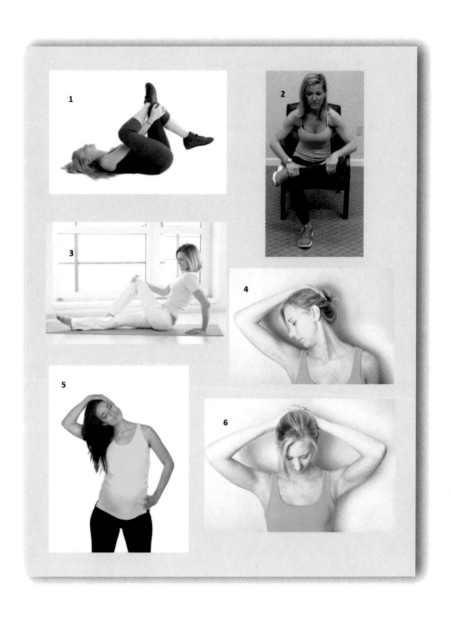

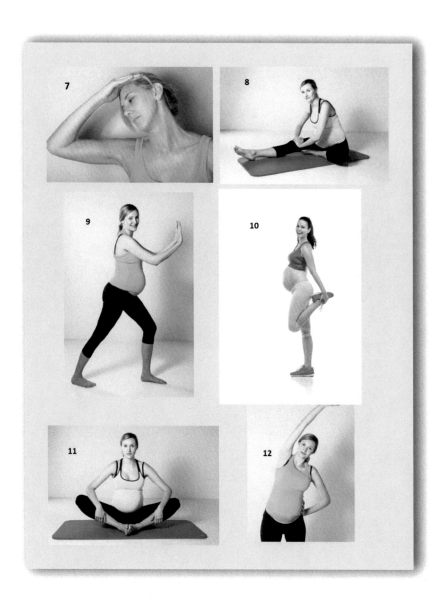

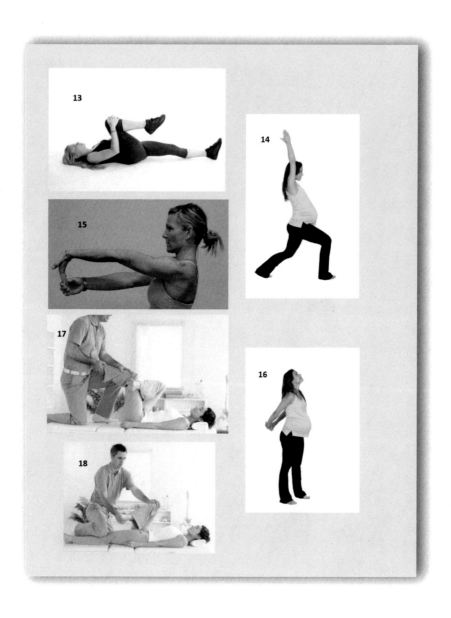

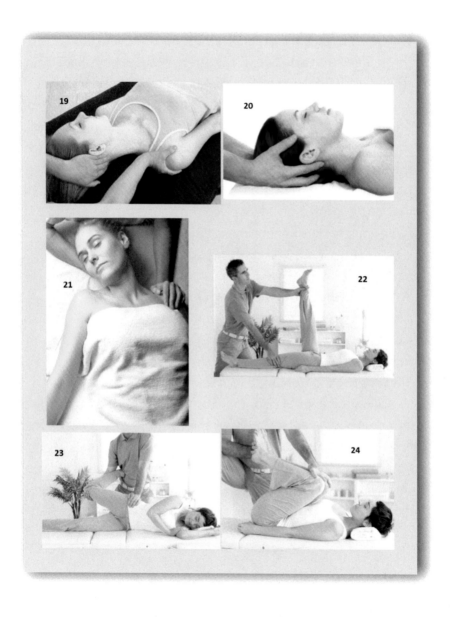

Prenatal Self-Stretching

Hold each stretch for twenty to thirty seconds, and repeat each three times on each side. If the stretch causes any sharp pain, stop. Stretch until you feel tension in the muscle and not pain. If you experience any numbness, tingling, nausea, or shortness of breath during any stretch that requires you to be on your back, then immediately stop and change positions, and get up when the symptoms subside. These symptoms may indicate an interruption of proper blood flow. Stretches performed on the back may be performed on a bed or on the floor—but be sure to use a yoga mat for cushioning if you choose the floor.

Stretch One: Piriformis Lying Down

After thirty weeks stop all stretching on your back. If you feel nauseous, dizzy, or faint while on your back, immediately turn to either side, and rest until the feeling passes, and switch to a different variation of the stretch such as seated.

Lie on the floor or bed, and cross your right leg over your left knee. Pull both knees toward your chest with your back flat on the floor or bed. Once you feel tension in your right buttock region, hold that pressure for twenty seconds. You can adjust how hard you are pulling the right (top) leg; this will slightly change where you feel the stretch in the right buttock. Repeat three times on both sides.

Stretch Two: Piriformis Seated

Sit with your hips slightly higher than your knees. Keep your back straight. Cross the left leg over the right leg so that your left ankle is resting on your right knee. Grasp your left knee with both hands, and pull it toward your chest with your left ankle still resting on your right knee until you feel tension in your left hip or buttock region. You can lean forward with a straight back and upright head to increase the tension. If the baby is in the way, lean slightly to the right to give more room. Hold for thirty seconds, and repeat three times on both sides.

Stretch Three: Glutes

After thirty weeks stop all stretching on your back. If you feel nauseous, dizzy, or faint while on your back, immediately turn to either side, and rest until the feeling passes, and switch to a different variation of the stretch such as seated.

Lie on your back or sit on the floor with your right leg out straight and your left leg bent at the knee. Cross your left leg across the right, and pull your left knee toward your chest and right shoulder until you feel tension in your left buttock region. You can pull it with your right hand. Stop and hold the stretch once you feel a stretch in the buttock region or lower back. Hold for thirty seconds. Do this stretch on the other side. Repeat three times on both sides.

Stretch Four: Levator Scapula

Sit or stand, and hold something with your left hand to keep your left shoulder down (for example, a two- to five-pound hand weight or a can of soup). Do not let your shoulder pop up during the stretch. Turn your head toward your right side to look over your right shoulder, and using your right hand, gently pull your head down toward your right hip until you feel tension in the left side of your neck and into your left shoulder blade. Hold for thirty seconds. Repeat on the other side. Do this three times on both sides.

Stretch Five: Upper Trapezius

Sit or stand, and hold something with your left hand to keep your left shoulder down (for example, a two- to five-pound hand weight or a can of soup). Do not let your shoulder pop up during the stretch. Turn your head toward your left shoulder, and gently pull your head forward with your right hand (so that you are looking up and out to the left) until you feel tension in the left side of your neck and into your left shoulder blade. Hold for thirty seconds. Repeat on the other side. Do this three times on both sides.

Stretch Six: Suboccipitals (base of head)

Sit or stand. Keep your head facing straight ahead. Tuck your chin to your chest, and gently pull your head forward with the weight of one or both hands. You should feel tension at the base of your head. Hold for thirty seconds, release and rest for 20 seconds, and repeat three times.

Stretch Seven: Scalenes

Sit or stand, and hold something with your left hand to keep your left shoulder down (for example, a two- to five-pound hand weight or a can of soup). Do not let your shoulder pop up during the stretch. Turn your head slightly to the right, and with your right hand, gently pull your head to the right side and slightly backward so your right ear goes toward your right shoulder. You should feel tension in the left front side of your neck. If you get any neck pain in the back or on the right side, do not pull back at all, only to the right. Hold for thirty seconds, and repeat with your left hand on the left side. Do this three times on both sides.

Stretch Eight: Hamstrings

Sit on the floor with your right leg out straight. Bend your left leg at the knee so that your left foot touches your right inner thigh. Keep your torso upright and your back straight, and lean forward, leading with your chest toward your right foot, until you feel tension in the back of your right leg. Keep your hips, right knee, and right foot straight ahead. Do not round your shoulders forward—keep them back and down. You can pull your toes backward to increase the stretch. Hold for thirty seconds. Repeat three times on both sides.

Stretch Nine: Calf

Stand straight, facing a wall. You can support yourself with your hands against the wall. Extend your right leg backward while keeping it straight and put your foot flat on the ground. Do not rotate your foot. Keep your leg straight, and lean forward until you feel tension in your right calf. Hold for thirty seconds. Repeat with the right knee slightly bent. Do this three times on both sides.

Stretch Ten: Quadriceps

Stand near a wall, and stabilize yourself with your right hand on the wall. Slowly lift your left heel, bringing it back toward your left buttock, and grab it with your left hand when you can. Alternatively, you can put your instep up on a stool and sit back. You should feel tension in the front of your left thigh. Hold for thirty seconds, and repeat three times on each side.

Stretch Eleven: Adductors

Sit on the floor. Keep your torso upright. Bring your feet together and close to your pelvis, and let your knees fall to each side. Let the weight of your legs pull your legs apart. Hold for thirty seconds, and repeat three times. You can increase the tension by gently pressing down on your knees with your elbows. Do not slouch.

Stretch Twelve: Quadratus Lumborum (QL)

Stand upright, reach your right arm up to the sky, and then slowly lean to the left until you feel tension in the right side of your back and rib cage. Hold for thirty seconds, and repeat on the other side. Do this three times on both sides.

Stretch Thirteen: Spinal Erectors (Lower Back)

    a. Lying down: Do not do this exercise lying down after thirty weeks. If you feel nauseous, dizzy, or faint while on your back, immediately turn to either side, and rest until the feeling passes, and do not do this stretch on your back again. Lie on the floor on your back. Pull one knee to your chest until you feel a comfortable stretch in the lower back and buttocks. Keep your back and neck relaxed. Hold for thirty seconds, and repeat three times with each knee.

b. Seated: Sit with your hips higher than your knees. Your knees will need to be wide apart. Rest your arms on your thighs. Slowly bend forward, allowing the baby and your torso to go between your legs. Picture your low-back curvature reversing, and once you feel a pull or stretch in the lower back, hold for thirty seconds. Then, slowly return to the starting position, using your arms to help push you back up to a neutral position. Repeat three times.

Stretch Fourteen: Hip Flexors

Stand with feet together. Take a large step forward with the right foot and keep the left foot stationary. Keep your pelvis, hips, and feet all pointing straight ahead. Do not let your pelvis rotate or your feet point out. Tighten your lower abdominals, and lift the baby up and back. Hold the abdominals as tight as possible, and then bend the right knee and slowly lunge forward until you feel tension in the front of your left hip or lower abdominal region. If you feel any pain in the lower back, try to tighten your lower abdominals harder to lift the baby higher. If you continue to have lower back pain, then shorten the distance between your feet to decrease the tension. Hold this for thirty seconds, and then repeat on the right side. Do this three times on each side. You can increase the tension by raising your hands straight up in the air at the same time as you lunge.

Stretch Fifteen: Forearm Flexors
Straighten your left arm with the palm facing the ceiling in front of you at shoulder height, as if you just threw a bowling ball. Keeping your elbow straight, use your right hand to pull your fingers down and back toward your body, so your fingers point toward the floor. You should feel tension anywhere from your fingers to your elbow. Hold for thirty seconds, and repeat three times on each side.

Stretch Sixteen: Pectoralis
While standing, bring your hands behind you, and interlock your fingers. Pull your shoulders down and back until you feel a comfortable stretch across your chest. Hold for thirty seconds, and repeat three times. You can look up toward the sky at the same time to increase the tension, if doing so does not cause pain in your neck.

Partner Stretching
If you get any numbness, tingling, nausea, or shortness of breath while doing any exercise on your back, immediately stop, change

positions, and get up when symptoms subside. Stretches performed on your back may be performed on a bed or on the floor—but be sure to use a yoga mat for cushioning if you choose the floor.

As your body progressively changes during your pregnancy, it will become increasingly challenging to stretch and care for yourself. Having a partner to help you can be very valuable, and your partner can feel empowered to take an active role in helping you manage your ever-changing body.

Stretch Seventeen: Piriformis

Lie on the floor or a bed, and cross your right leg over your left knee. Have your partner gently push both your right and left knees toward your chest, while you stay flat on your back. Once you feel tension in your buttock region, have your partner hold that pressure for twenty seconds. Repeat three times on both sides. Once you feel tension, your partner can adjust how hard he or she is pushing your right (top) leg; this will slightly change where you feel the stretch.

Stretch Eighteen: Glutes

Lie on your back with your right knee drawn toward your chest. Have your partner slowly push your bent right leg across your body, toward your left shoulder. Stop and hold once you feel a stretch in the buttock region or lower back. Hold for thirty seconds. Repeat three times on each side.

Stretch Nineteen: Levator Scapula and Upper Trapezius

Lie down with your head at the end of a bed on a pillow. Turn your head toward your left side, and have your partner gently use his or her right hand to press your right shoulder down while lifting your head forward with the left hand until you feel tension in the neck or shoulder blade region. Hold for thirty seconds, and repeat three times on both sides.

Upper Trapezius: Repeat the levator scapula stretch (19), but turn your head toward the right side, and have your partner gently use his or her right hand to press your right shoulder down and lift your head forward with the left hand until you feel tension in the neck and shoulder blade region. Hold for thirty seconds, and repeat three times on both sides.

Stretch Twenty: Suboccipitals

Lie down with your head at the end of a bed on a pillow. Look at the ceiling. Gently tuck your chin to your chest, and have your partner gently lift your head forward until you feel tension in the neck and shoulder blade region. Hold for thirty seconds, and repeat three times.

Stretch Twenty-One: Scalenes

Lie down with your head at the end of a bed on a pillow. Turn your head toward the right side, and have your partner gently use his or her left hand to press your left shoulder down and the right hand to guide your neck to the right until you feel tension on the left side of the front of the neck. Hold for thirty seconds, and repeat three times on both sides. Be very gentle with this stretch, and stop if it is painful.

Stretch Twenty-Two: Hamstrings

Lie on your back, and tighten and flatten your lower back to the floor. Have your partner gently and slowly lift your left leg while you keep it straight. Stop when you feel tension on the back of your leg. Hold for thirty seconds. Repeat three times on each side.

Stretch Twenty-Three: Quadriceps and Hip Flexors

Lie on your side with two pillows between your legs. Position the pillows lengthwise so that your entire leg is supported from the groin to the ankle. Have your partner stand behind you, lift your knee up, and gently pull your foot and knee back toward your buttocks until you feel a stretch on the front of your thigh. If you experience any lower back pain, stop, or decrease the tension. Hold for thirty seconds. Repeat three times on both sides.

Stretch Twenty-Four: Spinal Erectors (Lower Back)

Lie on the floor on your back. With your hands behind your knees, have your partner push both knees toward your chest or abdomen until you feel a comfortable stretch in the lower back and buttocks. Keep your back and neck relaxed. Hold for thirty seconds, and repeat three times. If it is not possible to do this later in the pregnancy, try the seated self-stretch seventeen.

Partner stretching and massage can be great ways for the other parent or partner to become actively involved in helping you enjoy a happy pregnancy. Often a partner feels helpless and frequently is looking for a way to play a more important role and bond with you and the baby.

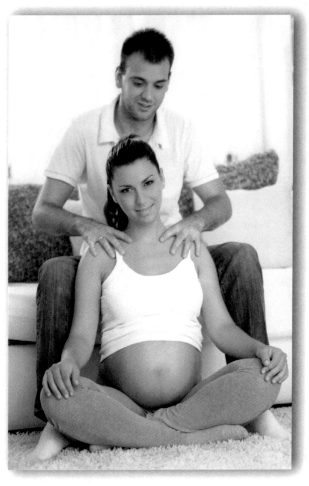

Partner Massage

First, contact your health care provider to find out whether partner massage is safe for you. After you've been cleared by your provider, find a position that is comfortable for you, either lying on your side or seated:

- Side lie position—lie on your side on a yoga mat on the floor or on a firm bed, with one or two pillows between your legs and a pillow under your head.
- Sitting position—sit in a chair with a comfortable backrest so your hips and knees are parallel, or sit on the floor with your partner behind you.

Have your partner use gentle strokes and alternate large and small circular motions. He or she should not put pressure on any hard bony prominences, such as the midline of the spine. Focus on your feet, calves, hips, back, neck, and shoulders. A daily ten-minute foot massage can help a lot. Coconut oil can be used after the first trimester as a great massage oil.

Keep these cautionary tips in mind:

- Do not use massage oil or essential oil until after the first trimester.
- Do not put any pressure on the abdomen.
- Drink a large glass of water after each massage.
- Stay clear of pressure points on the wrists and ankles, as these may induce contractions.

- Do not do deep tissue massage. Always use gentle strokes.
- Stop immediately if you experience any pain, dizziness, nausea, or other abnormal sensations.

Icing

Ice is best applied when standing or lying down rather than when sitting. Your hip flexors will tend to tighten if you sit to ice. Never apply the ice pack directly to the skin—be sure to have a barrier between your skin and the ice pack. You can place it between your underwear and compression-type shorts or leggings for the same type of barrier. You can also lie on your side in the pregnancy sleeping position and ice there. You can ice for fifteen–twenty minutes, wait at least thirty minutes, and then reapply the ice. Common areas to ice are the sacroiliac or low-back regions, feet, neck, and hips.

Rehab Exercises For Home Care

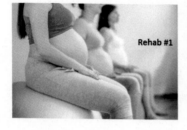
Rehab #1

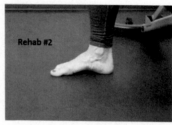
Rehab #2

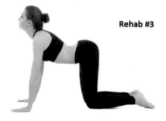
Rehab #3

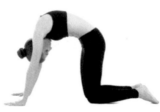

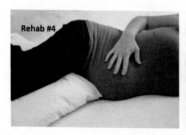
Rehab #4

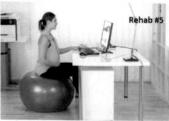
Rehab #5

Home Rehab Exercises and Postures

Here is a list of home rehab exercises and postures to use as part of your home care for the conditions section of this book. Active participation is critical for your overall health care success.

Exercise One: Physioball Seated Posterior Pelvic Tilt

Inflate your physioball to the height at which your hips are slightly higher than your knees when you sit on it. Most women will need a sixty-five centimeter ball. Sit on the ball. You can find center by gently bouncing up and down until you can almost lift your legs off the ground and be balanced. Stop bouncing. Begin the exercise by tightening your lower abdominal muscles and using the muscles to lift your baby up and back. This will naturally tuck your tailbone underneath you. Make sure to keep your torso upright and your head and shoulders back and down. Do not slouch. The ball should not move much. Relax, and return to the starting positon. You can exhale as you tighten your abdominals and inhale as you return to the starting position. You can also try to tighten your pelvic floor muscles at the same time as you tighten your lower abdominals. This should be a very comfortable exercise and should not cause any pain. Keep your hips higher than your knees and your knees and feet straight ahead and hip width apart. As you get into the late stages of your third trimester, you may need to spread your knees apart more. Hold the contracture for a couple of seconds, and then relax. Repeat this ten times, and do three sets of ten total. You can also sit and do gentle clockwise and counterclockwise circles on the ball.

See picture of rehab exercise 1.

Exercise Two: Toe Curls

Sit in a chair with your hips slightly higher than your knees. Keep your hips, knees, and feet all facing straight ahead and your feet hip width apart. Imagine your feet being hands, and curl the bottoms of your feet, and make a fist with your toes. Hold it for two seconds, and then relax. Repeat this ten times, and do three sets of ten repetitions. Rest for one minute between each set. It is common for the bottoms of your feet to cramp when you are starting this. If they do, massage them or roll them over a tennis or golf ball to loosen them up.

See picture of rehab exercise 2.

Exercise Three: Cat and Camel

Get down on your hands and knees on the floor. Relax your head, and allow it to droop. Round your back up toward the ceiling until you feel a nice stretch in your upper, middle, and lower back. Hold this stretch for as long as it feels comfortable (about fifteen to thirty seconds). Return to the starting position with a flat back. Then, let your back sway by pressing your stomach toward the floor. Lift your buttocks toward the ceiling. Hold this position for fifteen to thirty seconds. Repeat two to four times.

See picture of rehab exercise 3.

Posture is often thought of as a passive activity and not given enough attention. Correct posture is key to decreasing stress to muscles and joints in order to allow them to recover from abnormal use. Actively maintaining a correct posture will also strengthen deconditioned key core muscles. Maintaining proper posture is an exercise that requires active mental and physical input. Changing posture is a gradual process that requires consistency.

Posture One: Sleeping

Use two pillows, on top of each other, between your knees and feet when you sleep on your side, and keep your knees parallel and legs straight. Do not bend them up to your chest. Tighten your lower abdominal muscles to lift the baby up and back before you roll over or try to get out of bed. Keep the pillows between your legs when you roll over in bed.

See picture of rehab exercise 4.

Posture Two: Sitting

Every thirty minutes, take a break from sitting to stand or stretch. Keep your hips higher than your knees. Do not sit cross-legged as this will cause your piriformis muscles to shorten. Keep your hips, knees, and feet facing straight ahead. Keep your elbows by your sides; do not reach forward for your keyboard or mouse. Stay close enough to your desk to keep your elbows by your side. Keep your elbows higher than your wrists, and keep your shoulders and head back. When you have the opportunity, elevate your feet with ice on them for twenty minutes to help with swelling but then return to the neutral sitting position.

See picture of rehab exercise 5.

Posture Three: Driving

Keep your hips higher than your knees. Keep your hips, knees, and feet facing straight ahead. Do not rotate either foot outward. Keep your elbows by your side. Use an underhand grip on the steering wheel, with your hands at eight and four o'clock to avoid reaching your arms forward and slouching your head and shoulders.

CHAPTER 9

Office-Based Care

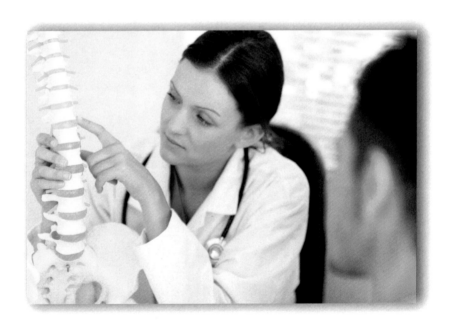

Chiropractic Joint Manipulation

Research has shown that chiropractic joint manipulation uniquely relaxes the pelvic floor muscles during the second trimester in preparation for delivery. This may decrease the chances of vaginal tearing during the delivery.

Many chiropractic physicians, including those on the Hemmett Health team, use motion palpation to assess for proper joint motion in every joint in the body. Various factors can contribute to abnormal or restricted joint motion. Acute trauma, such as whiplash, or prolonged or repetitive abnormal stress, such as from habitual poor posture or poor posture from pregnancy, stresses the ligaments and muscles surrounding the joints.

Joint motion restrictions cause friction and increased stress on the normal joint function. This increased friction may cause inflammation, pain, or just joint wear and tear.

This wear and tear is no small matter. Wear and tear can cause osteoarthritis, which is a progressive breakdown of cartilage. This cartilage is a very thin layer inside the joint. Thus, it becomes very important to remove stress from the joint in order to prevent complete degeneration of the cartilage.

Once a restricted joint has been located, a very specific force is exerted into the joint axis in order to restore the proper joint motion. This force, or thrust, is called a joint manipulation or adjustment. The thrust stimulates mechanoreceptors in the joint and relieves pain and reduces muscle spasm. These mechanoreceptors decrease pain signals, resulting in muscle relaxation.

It is very important to restore joint function if you are experiencing pain or disability as a result of these joint restrictions, particularly if you have been experiencing repeated or prolonged episodes of pain or disability. Repeated episodes often lead to chronic problems that affect the surrounding structures (joint capsules, ligaments, muscles, nerves, etc.).

Hold-Relax Post Neuromuscular Facilitation (PNF)

PNF is used to facilitate the relaxation of muscles to increase your range of motion. This technique can be more effective at increasing range of motion than stretching alone. The body part is put in a pain-free position, and then you contract the muscle that we want to stretch while your provider resists your push so you do not move the body part at all. You then relax the muscle, and your provider moves the body part to a new pain-free position. This hold-relax method of PNF takes advantage of Golgi tendon neurological reflexes to facilitate relaxation of the muscle and increased range of motion.

Active Release Techniques (ART)

ART is a soft-tissue therapy that diagnoses and treats soft-tissue (muscle, ligament, nerve, and fascia) restrictions and adhesions. It is sort of like massage, stretching, and trigger-point work all rolled up into one with the patient being moved or moving him- or herself through a full range of motion. You get the hurts-so-good feeling. The goal of ART is to restore normal tissue tension and tone, lengthening muscles and fascia to decrease localized pain and inflammation, either acute or chronic. ART can be a stand-alone therapy or used in conjunction with chiropractic joint manipulation.

Graston Technique

The Graston technique is a form of instrument-assisted soft-tissue mobilization that enables providers to address scar tissue and fascial restrictions. The technique uses specially designed stainless steel instruments, along with appropriate therapeutic exercises, to specifically detect and effectively treat areas exhibiting soft-tissue fibrosis or inflammation.

Massage

Massage aids in muscle relaxation, relieves spasms, increases range of motion, stretches tissue, and positively affects certain scar tissue. Muscles benefit from massage directly from contact and indirectly from improved circulation. After a massage, the body can more efficiently circulate clean, oxygenated blood and discard deoxygenated blood and other wastes, such as lactic acid.

Healthy muscles are less likely to become injured. Massage improves flexibility and increases range of motion. It promotes circulation and lymph which may also decrease recovery time after strenuous activity, which can result in less soreness. It may also promote a positive self-image and enhance a general sense of well=being.

Ergonomics and Postural Training

Your health care provider should always work hard to find all the activities of daily living that will aggravate your pregnant body and seek to modify them to make them less irritating. He or she can assess your workstation setup, sleeping positions, and recreational activities in an effort to teach you good new habits and correct old bad habits. Adopting long-term lifestyle changes during pregnancy can even help prevent chronic degenerative issues in the future.

Rehabilitative Strengthening Exercises

Your health care provider should focus on helping you achieve and maintain a strong, stable core, neck, shoulders, and feet as early as possible and throughout the pregnancy, as well as during postnatal recovery. Most common prenatal orthopedic conditions involve an instability in one or more of these three regions. Adopting and maintaining high-quality strengthening exercises for the long term can have a very significant positive impact over your lifetime. Active rehabilitative strengthening exercises complement passive in-office therapies very well.

Custom-Molded Biomechanical Orthotics

The hyperpronation or flattening of the arch of the foot associated with pregnancy is best treated with a truly custom, biomechanically correct foot orthotic. Some research has shown that the changes in the way a woman walks during pregnancy may have a lasting effect and may not return to normal following birth. Some experts feel that the shoe size changes associated with flattening of the arch during pregnancy can be permanent in some women. Our providers use a custom full-foot, constant-contact, semirigid orthotic to raise your arch back up to its neutral position and thus shorten the foot back to its normal length.

CHAPTER 10

Conclusion

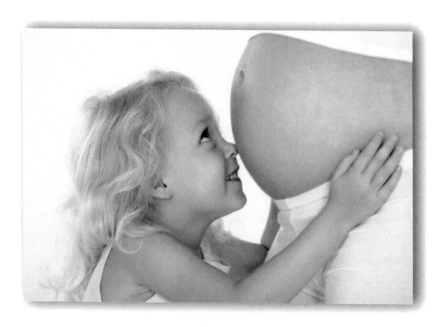

Please remember the instructions for using oxygen masks on airplanes: you must first put on your own mask before putting on your child's mask. The transition to parenthood is not easy. Parenthood will require you to work extra hard to take care of yourself so that you can take care of your family. Follow our recommended prenatal empowerment strategies to help prepare yourself to help your newborn baby.

If you do suffer from one or more orthopedic conditions prenatally, then make sure to follow up with your health care provider around the time of your six-week postnatal obstetrical appointment in order to determine the proper postnatal treatment plan. You can also read our next two books, *Postnatal Care* and *Pelvic Floor Care*, to find great self-help empowerment strategies as well as direction for in-office care. Please also read our book *Pediatric Orthopedic Care* to see how to prevent and treat some common injuries your new child may develop as he or she grows.

Parenthood is a wonderfully crazy and exciting journey. We hope to empower you to manage the many challenges to your body and the body of your growing baby with our three other books on postnatal care, pelvic floor care, and care for children. We hope you will enjoy reading them as much as we have enjoyed writing them and that you will use them as a resource and tool to help empower you to live a happy, healthy, and vibrant life. Visit our website, HemmettHealth.com, to purchase endorsed products and to view nutritious recipes and other gems.

Thank you for allowing us to be part of your health care team during this most exciting time. Please help empower other women who are taking this wonderful journey by sharing this book with them.

Warmly,

Drs. Vicki and Erik Hemmett

Reference List

Haddow, Watts, and Robertson J. 2005. "Effectiveness of a pelvic floor muscle exercise program on urinary incontinence following childbirth." *International Journal of Evidence Based Healthcare* May 3(5);103-46.

Morkved, and Bo K. 2014. "Effect of pelvic floor muscle training during pregnancy and after childbirth on prevention and treatment of urinary incontinence: a systematic review." British Journal of Sports Medicien48;299-310

Stergiakouli, Thapar, and George Davey Smith. 2016. "Association of Acetaminophen Use During Pregnancy With Behavioral Problems in Childhood." *Journal of American Medical Association Pediatrics* August 15, 2016. Doi:10.1001/jamapediatrics.2016.1775.

Please visit the 'Books' page at HemmettHealth.com for information about how to access our other books that will be published.

About the Authors

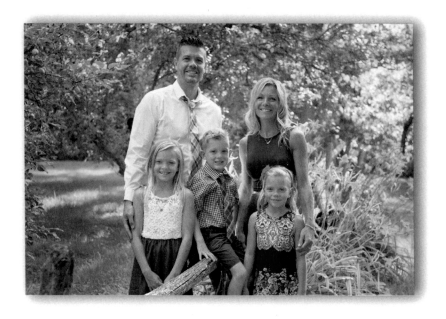

E very mother wants to do what is right for her child. This starts in the womb! Proper nutrition and simple exercises can help keep the mother-and thus the baby-happy, healthy and vibrant throughout pregnancy. Pregnancy doesn't have to bring debilitating pain and postnatal dysfunction. Chiropractic and prenatal experts Drs. Vicki and Erik Hemmett are here to help mothers alleviate aches and pains associated with pregnancy.

After receiving four-year bachelor's degrees, Drs. Vicki and Erik Hemmett both completed their doctor of chiropractic degrees from the National University of Health Sciences in Lombard, IL. Upon graduation in April 2002, they eagerly moved to Dr. Erik's native Vermont and purchased an existing practice in Willison. Together they grew the practice and in July 2008 they moved the practice to its current flagship location on Tilley Drive in South Burlington in the Eastern View Integrated Medical Building with Maitri Healthcare for Women OB-GYN practice and other integrative and collaborative practices.

Dr. Vicki has had tremendous success collaborating with a variety of medical providers to treat their perinatal patients and patients with pelvic floor conditions utilizing a combination of Hemmett Pelvic Floor Release Technique, chiropractic joint manipulation and rehab.

Dr. Vicki and Dr. Erik currently live in Richmond with their two daughters, Sienna and Quinn, and son, Reece. They all enjoy living a healthy active outdoor lifestyle together.